MW01680759

The Doctor Says I Have Kidney Disease Now What?

Written by Aaron G. Perry

Illustrated by Brandon Hadnot-walker

The Doctor Says I Have Kidney Disease Now What?

ISBN: 979-8-9890534-6-9

Illustrated by Brandon Hadnot-Walker

For more information on purchases in bulk, partnerships, or speaking events, please contact Aaron Perry at Ironmanaaron49@gmail.com or https://rebalanced-life.org/

The information provided within this book is for general informational and educational purposes only. Always consult a healthcare professional for your individual needs and for matters relating to your health and any symptoms that may require diagnosis or medical attention.

Kameron lay in the bed, reflecting on everything that happened over the last few months. He was in the trenches. He just couldn't get over how hard his life became.

Who would've imagined that so much would happen in such a short amount of time? More importantly, when would there finally be a moment to catch a breath? He then quietly shared a colloquial expression of hardship to himself.

"Man, life is lifing way too hard right now. When am I ever gonna get a break?"

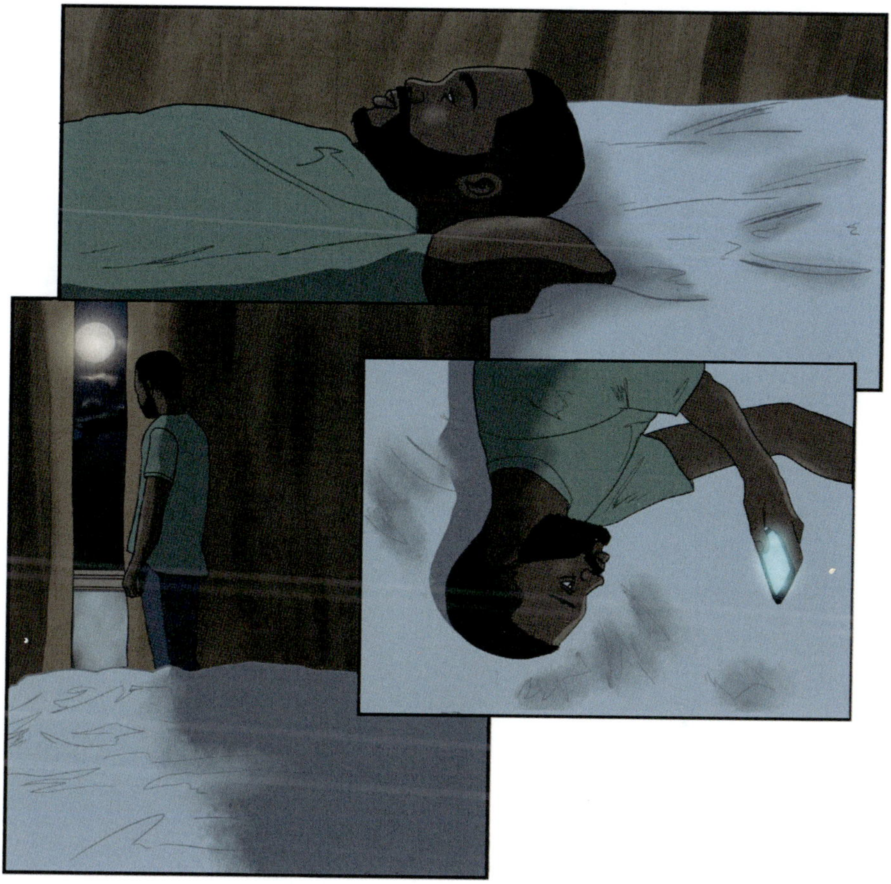

His pops, Uncle Cooley, as everyone called him, was still receiving care for colon cancer. His cousins Van and Ven were also dealing with their own struggles, all while expecting their first kids. Though they may as well have been his brothers, he didn't want to encumber them with his own issues. Kameron was emotionally dispersed; he was happy, scared, sad, and at times overwhelmed and confused. Life's hardships had taken a toll on him mentally and caused so much strain between him and Michele that she moved out.

The thick atmosphere of silence and tension in the household was suffocating her.

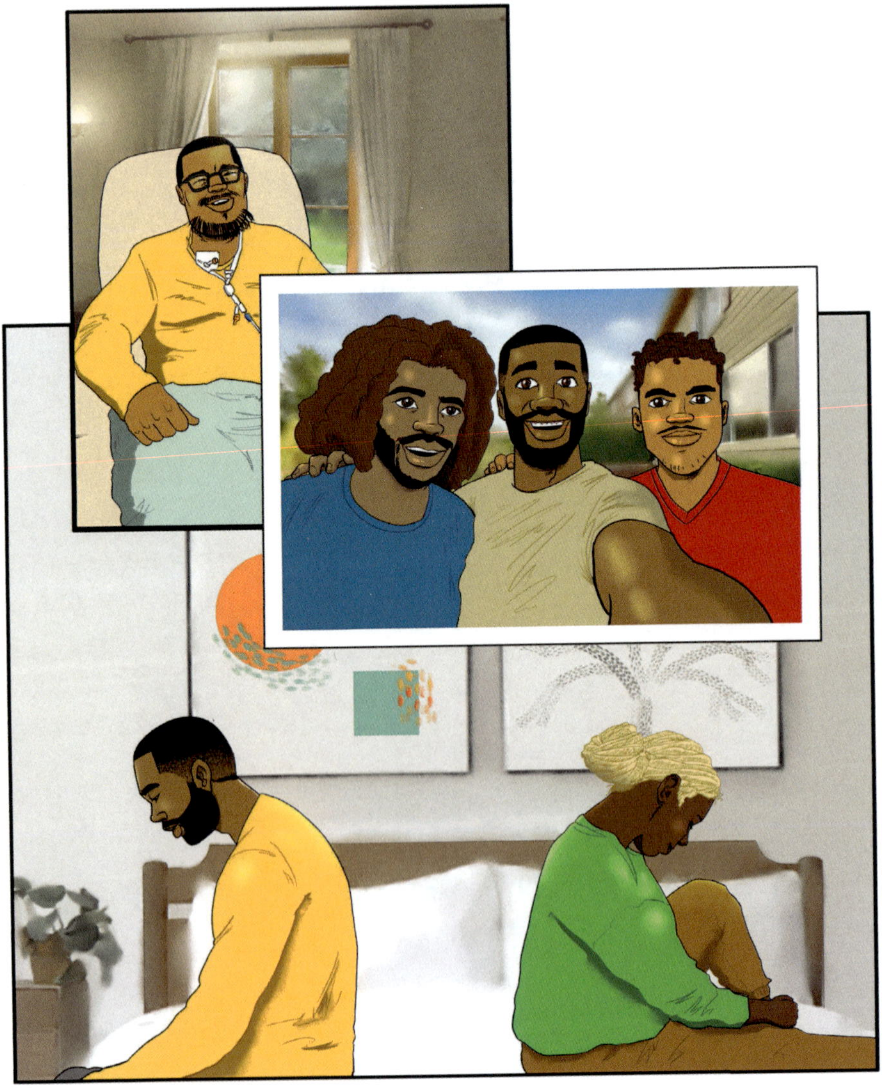

Michele repeatedly told Kameron how he's been mentally sporadic; remembering little-to-nothing concerning the details of their past conversations. Whenever they spoke, it seemed like he was a million miles away from her. After several small moments, her very last straw was discovering their serious conversation had become a monologue. Kameron was next to her, but he wasn't present.

After Michele stormed out, slamming the door behind her, he realized he'd drifted off, but it was far too late. The damage was done and he couldn't recall how long he'd been standing in that empty bathroom.

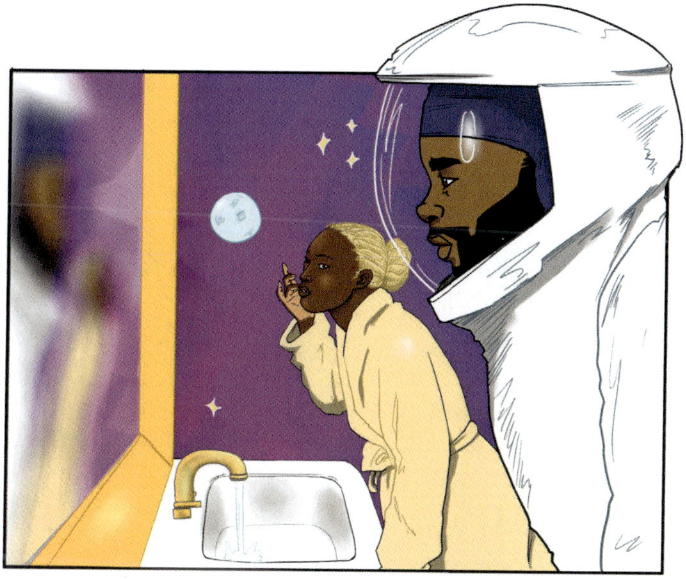

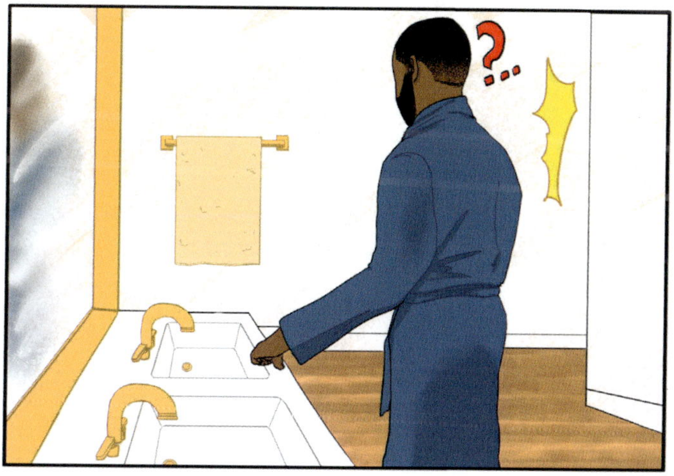

She left palpable fury in her wake. Every step a stomp, grumbled expletives unheard since their college days. She had chosen a path of internal peace and purity since then, which Kameron had now unintentionally disrupted. Things were escalating so fast, and with the speed at which her rage-fueled sentences flowed with clever strings of moderate disrespect... she'd put a battle rapper to shame. There was nothing he could do or say to stop her, and then his world went mute. She eerily calmed down and turned to him. Kameron saw Michele's lips move in slow motion to speak a nightmare into his reality.

"I think we just need a break." Michele dealt him a blow so heavy to the chest, it felt like he sank through the floor. As badly as he wanted to reply, it was like trying to stand perfectly still during a ravaging earthquake. Though he wanted to stop her, deep down in his heart, he figured time and space between the two of them might actually help.

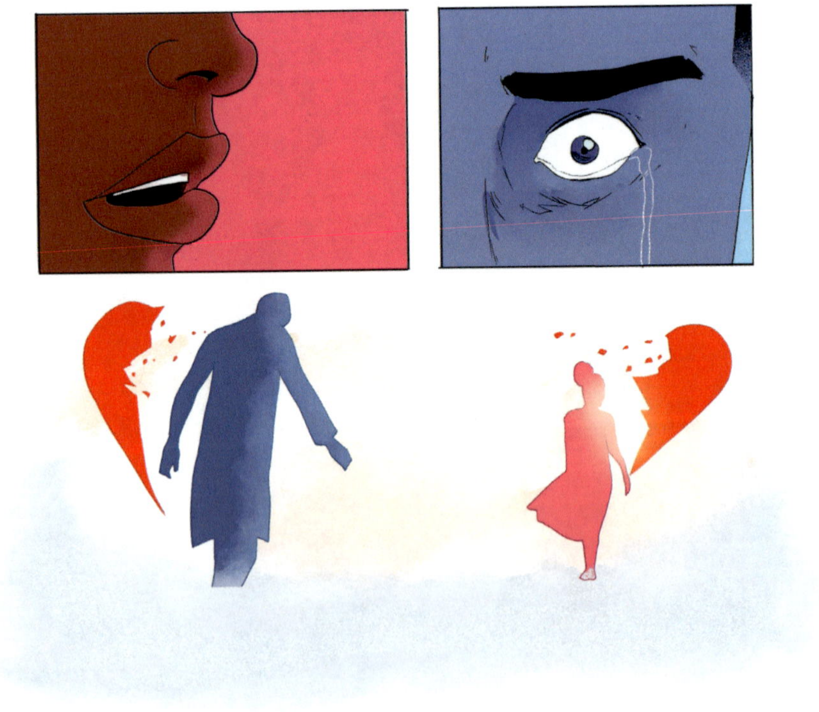

Kameron's phone pierced his state of conscience with a sharp ringing.

"Hey bro, what are you up to?" Van asked. "Not much, Just chilling," Kameron responded. There was an awkward silence.

"What's good, Cuzzo?" Kameron asked, breaking the awkward silence. "My dude, are you seriously going to act like you don't know where you are supposed to be right now?" Van responded, sounding a little aggravated.

"Huh?" Kameron replied, now starting to get irritated.

"Bro, you need to pull your head out of your butt. We have been talking about Black Men Run all week," Van responded fully irritated by what he felt was his disregard on Kameron's part.

"What? It's not Saturday!" Von responded. Why did Van always have to make everything a joke? This was so unfunny.

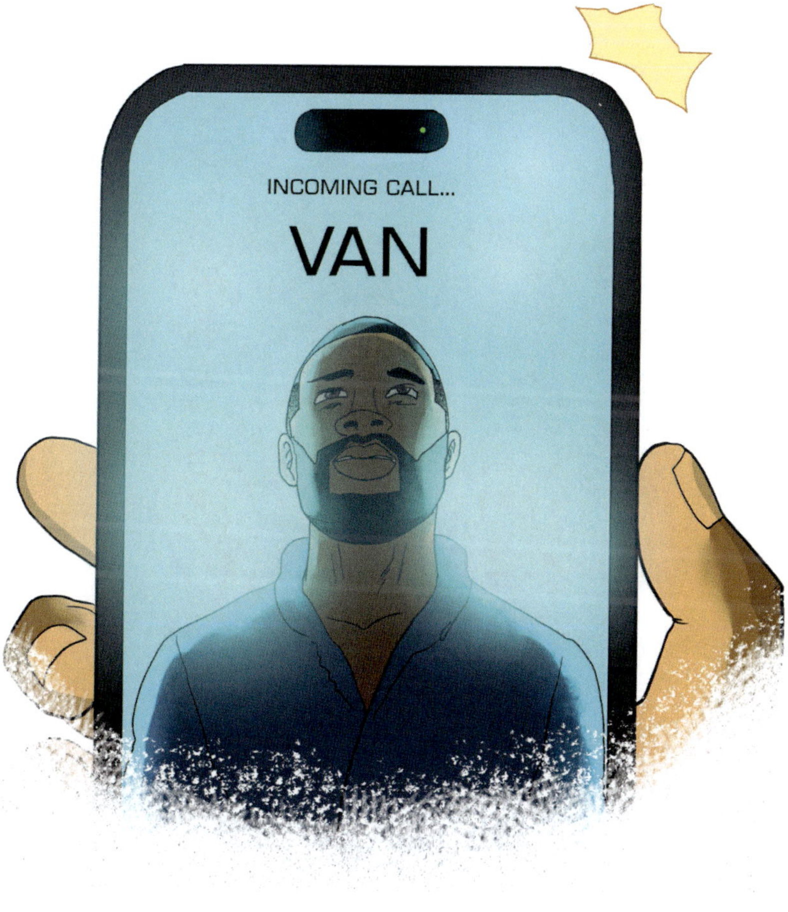

"If it's not Saturday, then I'm going to need another job and the group of men I am looking at, too," Van responded. "You coming, or naw?" Van asked.

"I'm in motion. I'm not that far from the spot. I'll catch up with y'all," Kameron responded with confusion. How did he lose two days? He was laying around and chilling about to get ready to head to work..." Did I go to work when I was supposed to?" He thought out loud to himself. Michele had always kept the calendar for the family. He shook this off as a fluke of not having Michele at home to keep him grounded.

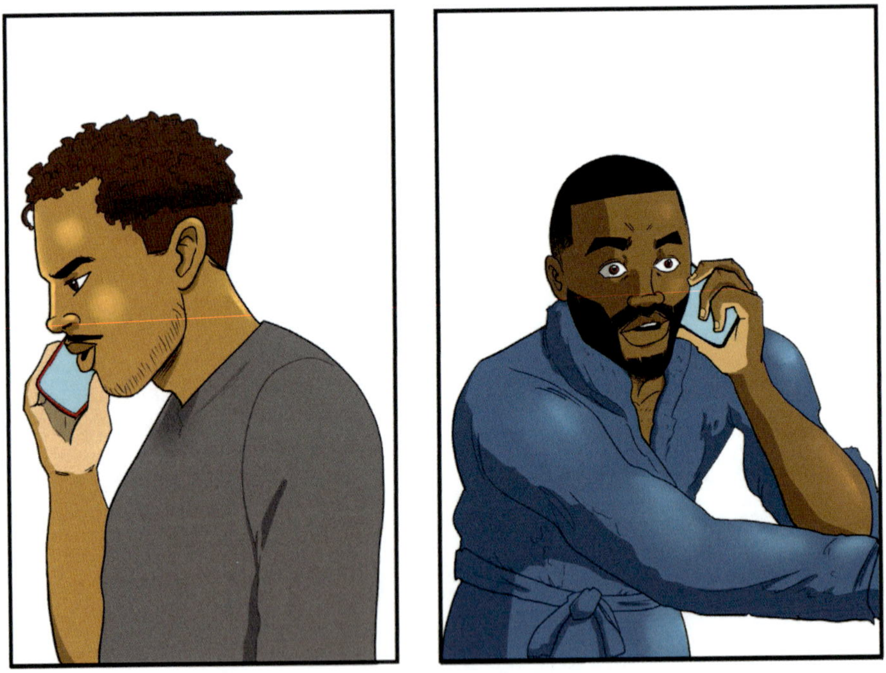

Kameron arrived at the site the men ran from and did a couple of quick stretches. He knew the route that the men generally took. He started sprinting to try and catch up with the group. As he was running he started to feel major spasms in his legs. He had to stop and walk. He tried drinking water, thinking maybe he was dehydrated. The spasms seemed to be replaced by an ache that felt like it was in the depths of his leg. It was odd and painful. He tried to walk it off, but it persisted. He then decided it may be best for him to return to the car.

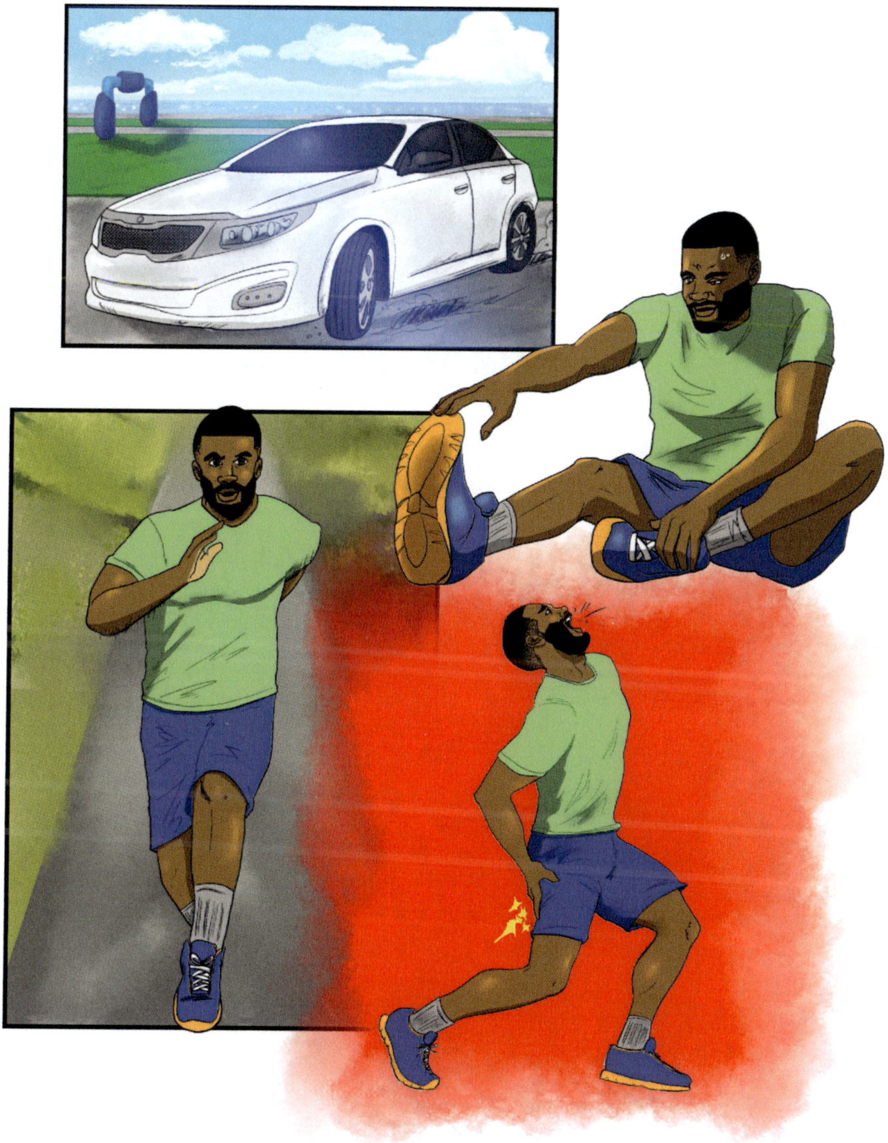

Kameron tried to keep moving once he arrived at the car, but the cramps were now accompanied by swelling in his ankles and hands. He sat down for a minute because he started to feel nauseous. He had heard so many people who had weird Covid symptoms.

"Do I have Covid?" He thought to himself. He wasn't sure what it was but he didn't want to take a chance of getting anyone else sick, so he sent Van and Ven a text and told them that he had come, but went home because he felt a little under the weather, not wanting anyone else to get sick.

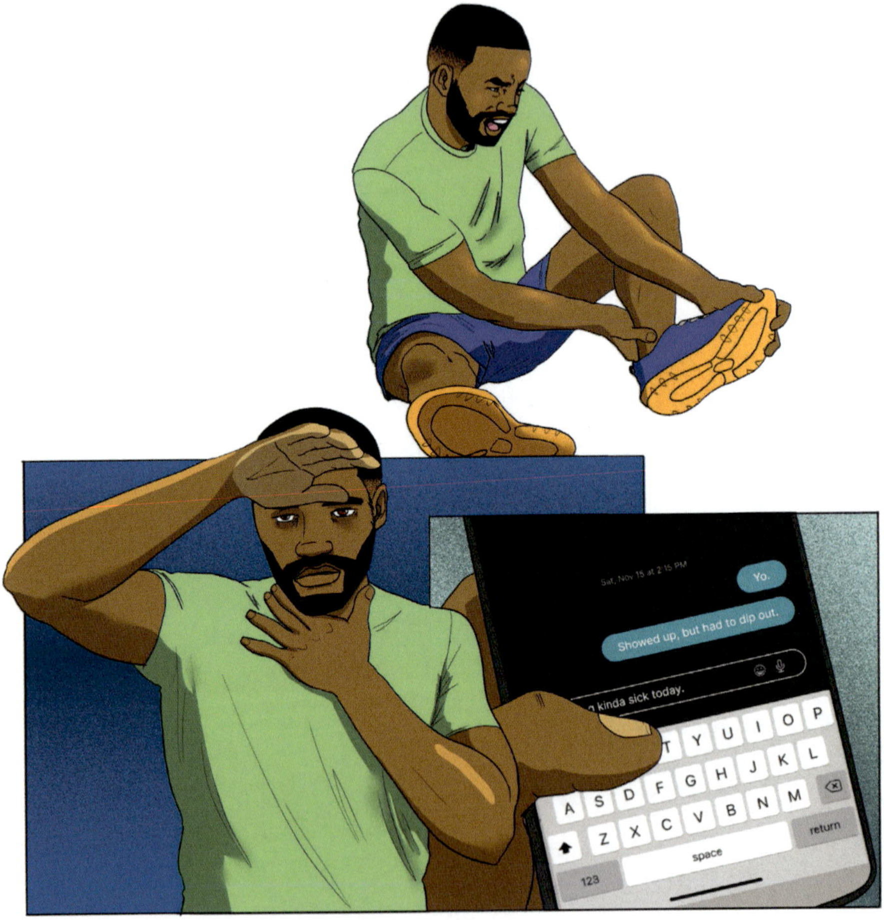

He got home and called Michele to tell her what was going on with him. She advised Kameron went to the emergency room. He told her that he was sure that he just needed to go take a nap. She opened her mouth to speak, but course-corrected her initial thought to avoid irritating him.

"Okay, Kam… but you have to call me if anything has changed."

Things had definitely changed. Through every sickness, Michele had been by his side and she didn't even offer to come over. He was tired and achy. He didn't feel like dealing with anyone in his space anyway. He went home, got in the bed, and went right to sleep.

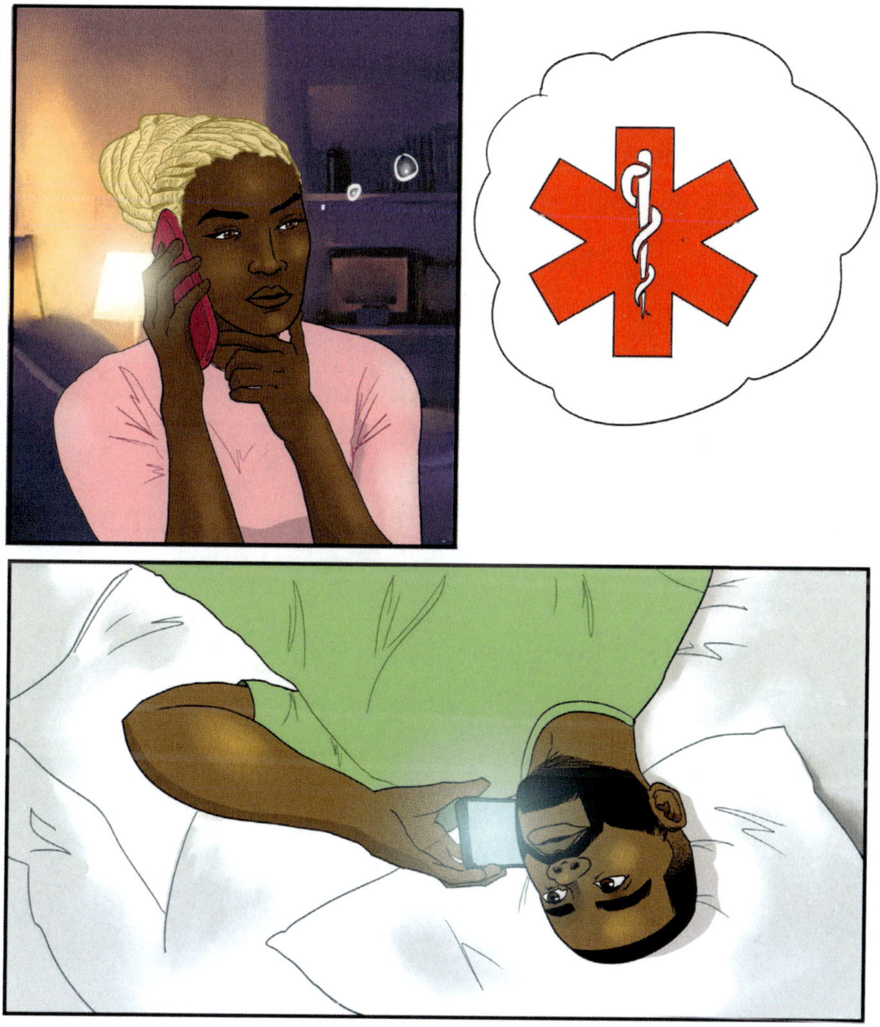

Suddenly, he woke up very disoriented. Kameron looked at his phone, reading 1:06 at the top of the lock screen.

It was dark outside his windows. He intended to take a nap only for a few hours, but he had slept the entire day away. Albeit strange, he shook it off and went into the kitchen to make a sandwich to settle his empty stomach. Then it dawned on him that he couldn't remember the last time he'd eaten. He took a few bites, but lost his appetite quickly.

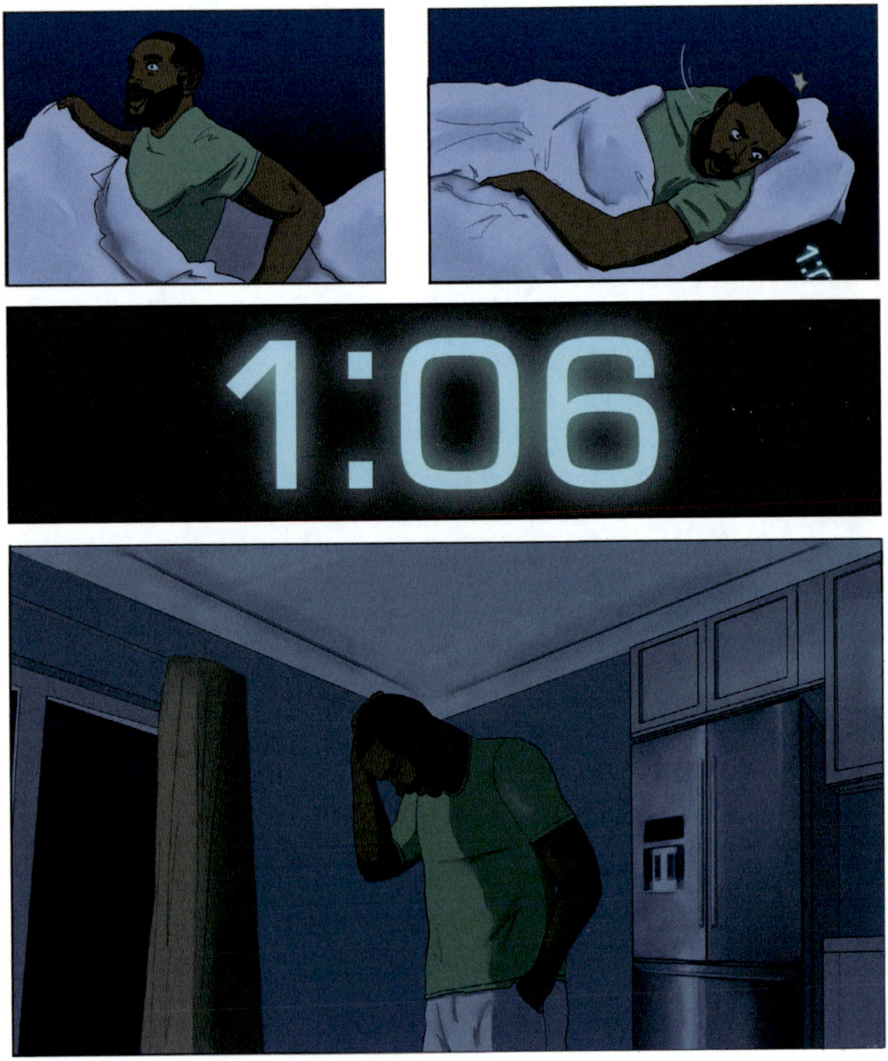

On returning to the bedroom after tidying up in the kitchen, Kameron picked up his phone. He had ten missed calls and forty-three texts. Most were from Van and Ven. It was far too late to call them, but Kameron shot out a quick text to let them know he went home and fell asleep.

Swiping through his notifications, he also missed a few calls and texts from Michele. Ringing Michele in wait for her sweet, but stern voice, was met by her voicemail. Another text to send as a quick status report so she wouldn't worry.

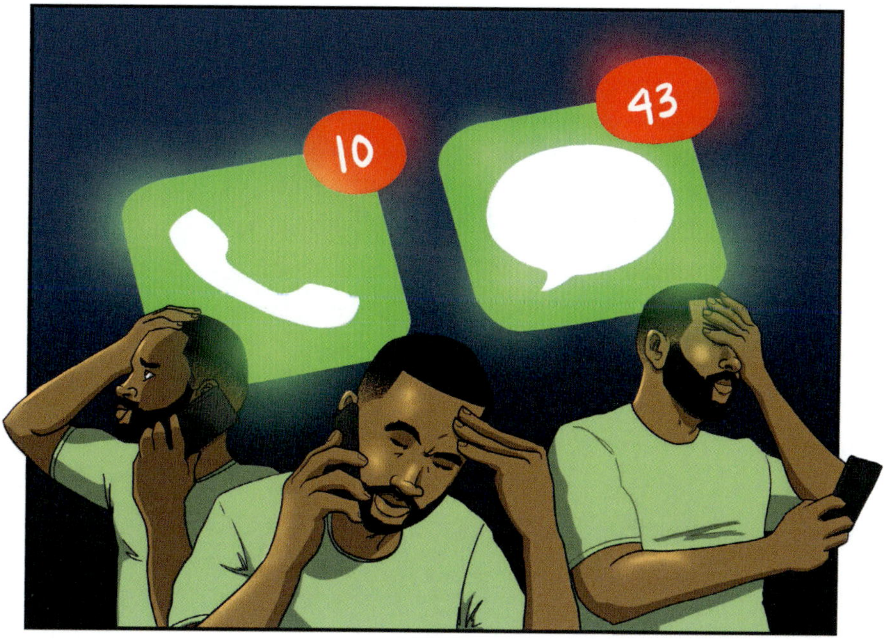

The phone buzzed loudly, causing Kameron to jump to attention. It was his father.

"Boy, what's goin' on with you?" His father, Pops, let his voice come in hot like it was the middle of the day.

"Hey, Pops…" Kameron tried to interject.

"Hey, Pops my #$@!," Uncle Cooley said with obvious irritation in his voice. "Boy, I'm going to ask you again, what is going on with you? Everybody and literally, their daddy, is calling me askin' about you. I got enough going on. You goin' through an early mid-life crisis?"

"Pops, c'mon." Kameron tried to get a word in.

"Pops, Pops, Pops, that's all you got to say? Don't even worry about it. I'll be over to see you in the morning. It's too late for this nonsense and I don't want to worry your Mama just 'cause she got a knuckle-headed son!" Pops swiftly ended the call.

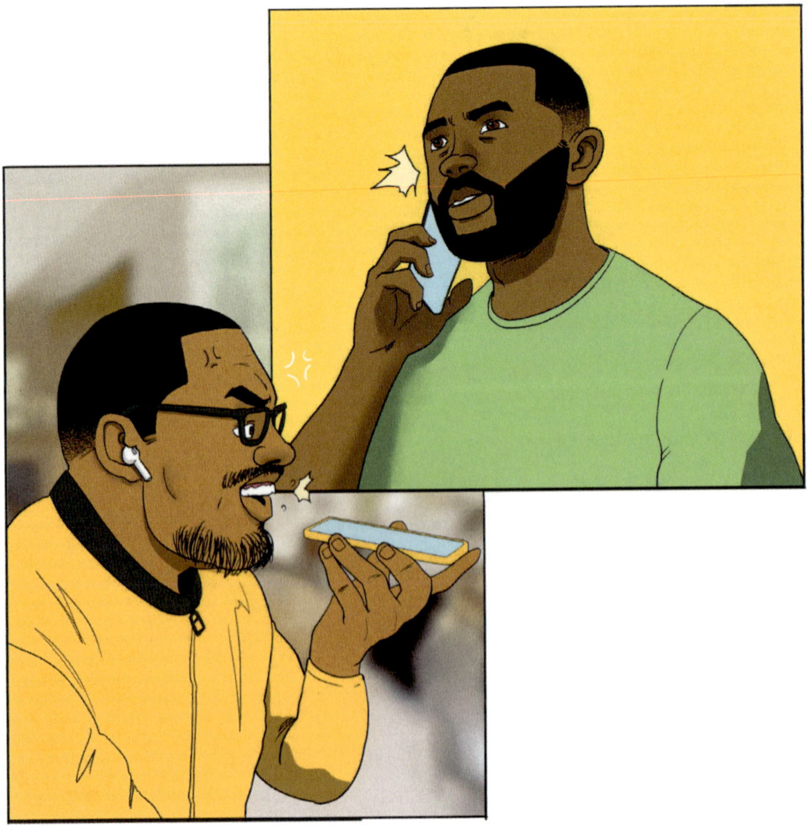

Kameron sat there looking at the phone. He laughed because Pops had always been that way when he was worried about him. Kameron couldn't understand why everyone was treating him like he had all of a sudden grown another head.

The weekend flew by. So did the next week.

Four Covid tests later and he was sure: he did not have the virus. Unfortunately, the fatigue, cramps, and lack of appetite continued.

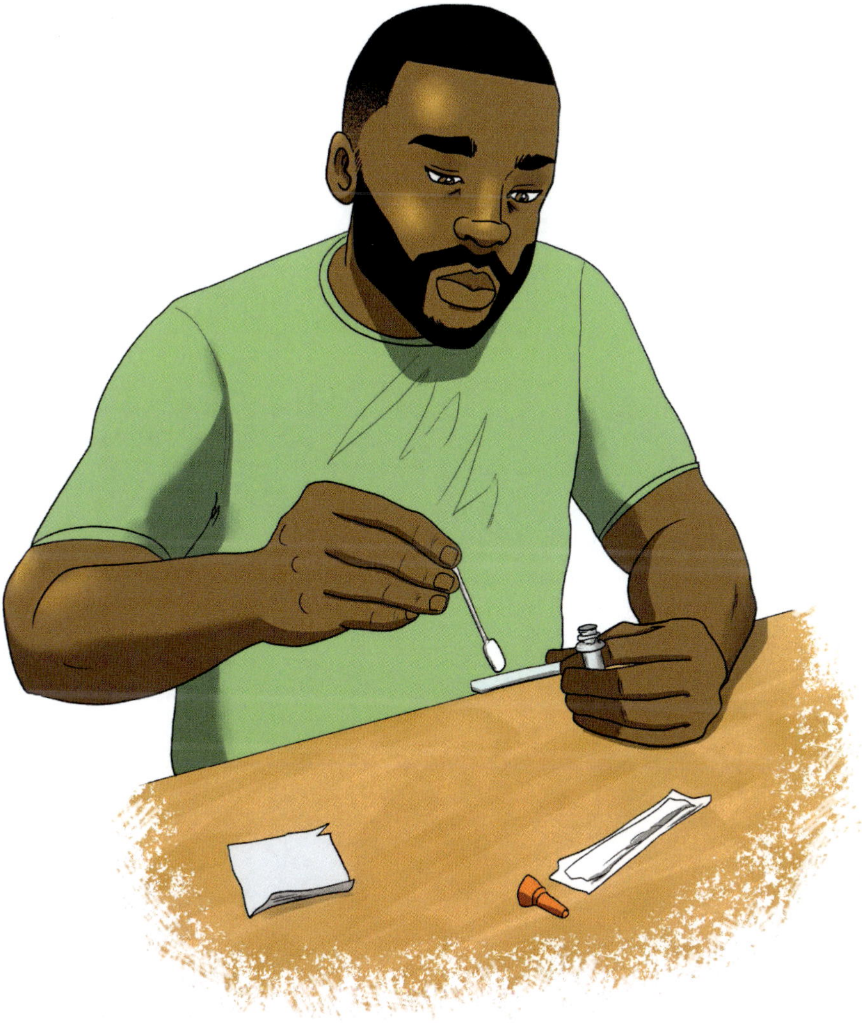

He met up at the barbershop with Van and Ven before the support group arrived, which Van and his dad facilitated regularly. They had just started to catch up with one another when the attention suddenly turned to Kameron.

“Aye, man… you’ve been MIA lately, you good?” Ven asked.

Kameron didn’t want the attention on him. He knew his dad would be arriving soon, so he didn’t want to get too deep into it.

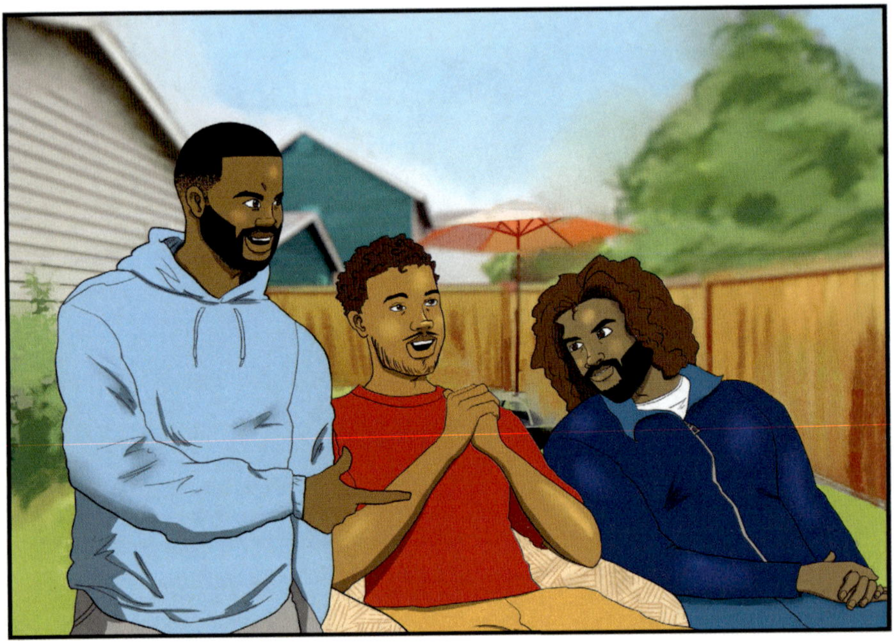

Uncle Cooley came in and gave everyone hugs, holding onto Kameron for a good minute. Everyone walked into the Rebalanced-Life Men's Center. Van and Uncle Cooley went into their Cancer Support Group. Ven scheduled to meet with his mental health professional at the time. Kameron decided to finally check in with a medical professional.

He went into the doctor's office and made small talk. The doctor obliged him for a little but then asked, "So, what really brought you into the office today?"

Kameron nervously twiddled his thumbs. "Everyone was doing their thing so I thought I'd just check in with someone."

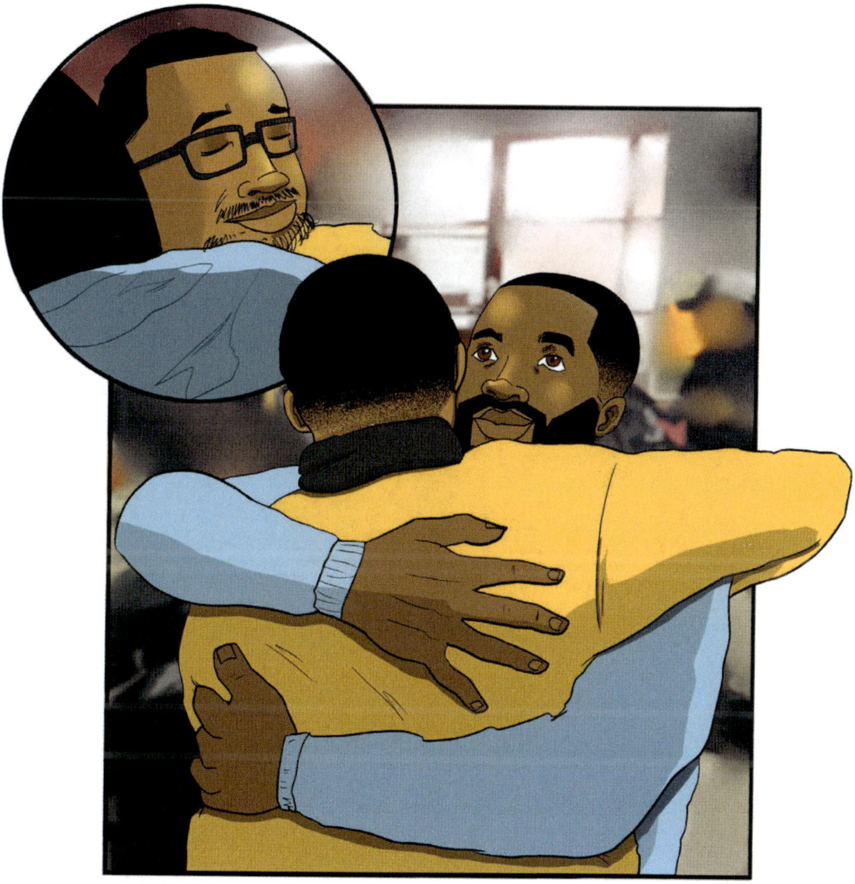

The doctor looked at Kameron intently.

"That's interesting. I know I've seen you around the shop before. We've spoken a number of times and you never just stopped in here. So, real talk this time, Kameron, what brought you in today?" Kameron looked at the doctor and hunched his shoulders.

Ultimately caving in, he listed off the things he was experiencing lately. He spilled everything: the loss of appetite, spasms, aches, lack of energy, swelling in his feet, and his struggle to focus, or pay attention.

"I should probably go and talk to Ven's therapist after we're done here, right?" Kameron said, followed by his forced laugh. The doctor recognized that he was worried and was trying his best to deflect.

"Well, Kameron, there could be a variety of reasons you are having these symptoms. So, we'll start with some tests. I'll order labs and we'll go from there," said the doctor in a caring tone.

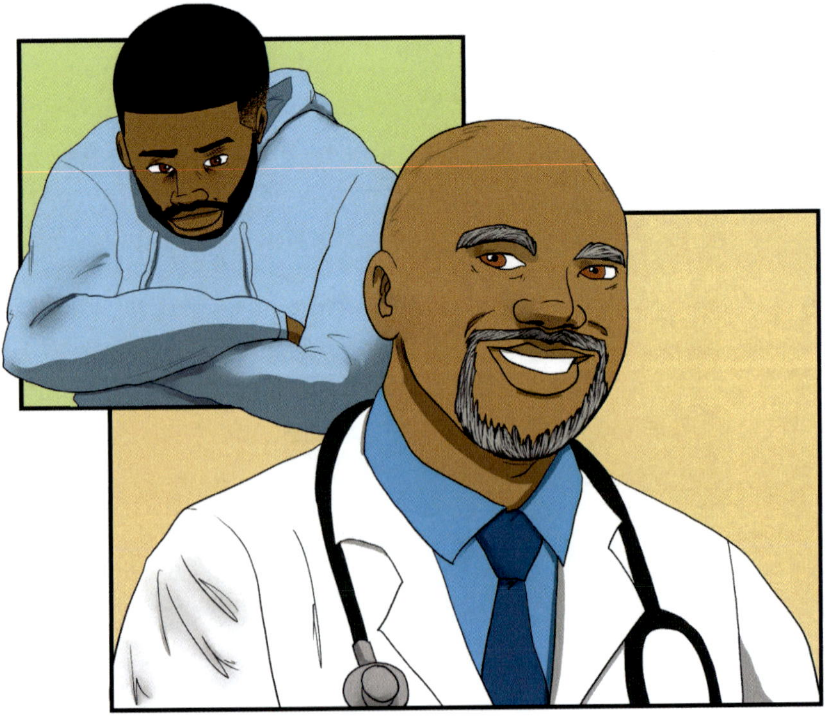

Kameron decided to get the tests done discreetly. After all, it could be nothing and there was no need to cause any of his loved ones to panic. Yet, he decided he was going to tell Michele, because she was still his wife, and even more despite the tension, still his friend.

Michele met him out at their restaurant. At first glance, Kameron noticed that she looked very different. He started to get nervous. Was there someone else? Was she fed up with this marriage? She was glowing with a honey-golden aura. His words were stuck in his mouth agape when he looked at her. She was somehow even more beautiful than he remembered, and he didn't think that was possible.

Michele looked at him and nervously smiled, "Boy, why are you looking at me like that?" Kameron was confused. He felt so many things: anger, fear, and confusion, to name a few.

"You look amazing. I guess this separation is working well for you." All of the weight of everything he'd been dealing with came out with his tone. He instantly regretted the words that escaped him without measure.

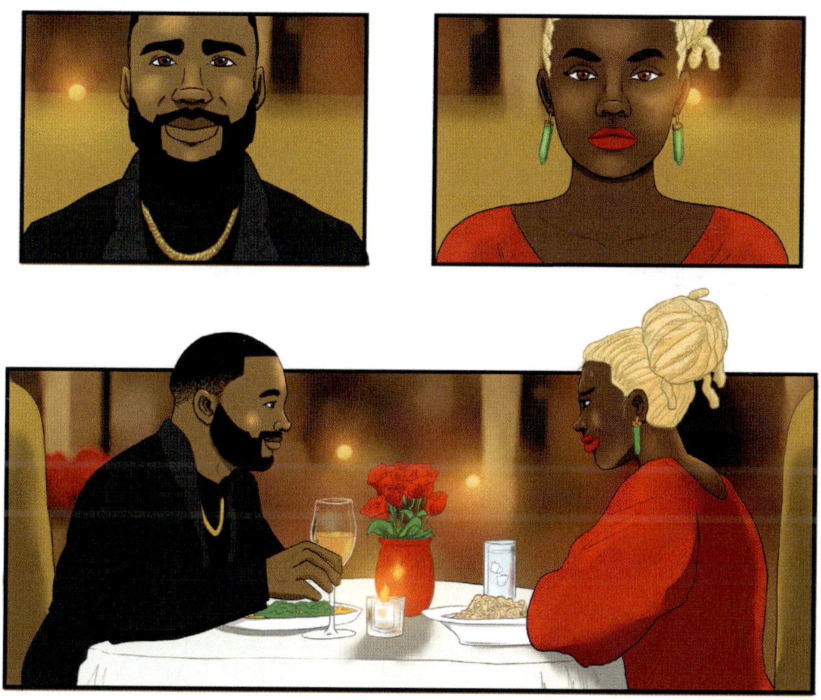

Michele turned away and sat quietly in her chair. She looked like she'd been hit by a heavy blow to the chest. Holding back tears of frustration, she sniffled and turned to him, "Look, I didn't come here to argue. We've done enough of that. You're either arguing with me or ignoring me. Speak your peace, Kam. I'm ready to go."

Kameron tried to fight back the tears that sprang to his eyes. He had never meant to hurt her, but that was all he seemed to do lately.

"Michele, I'm sorry," Kameron said. "I would never do anything ever to hurt you. You are the love of my life and I have missed you. I miss my friend most. It broke my heart the day I called you and told you that I wasn't feeling well, and you didn't seem to care. That was the first time since I met you that I have not had you with me when I was ill."

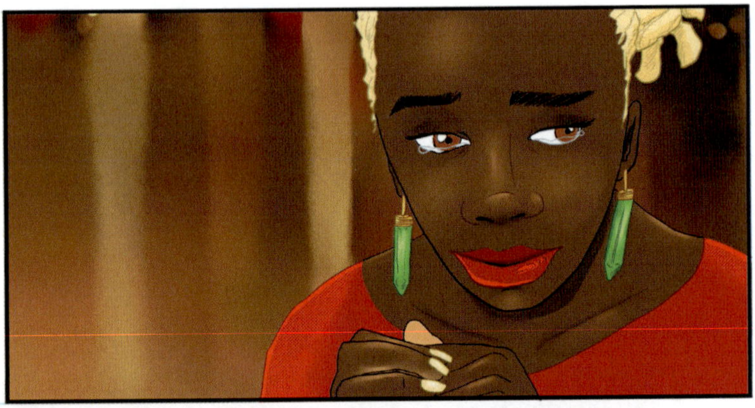

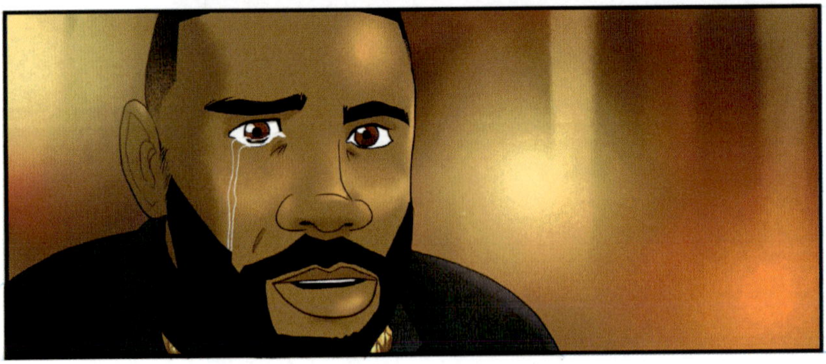

Michele was listening now, at least a little. She leaned forward and spoke in a softer voice of compassion.

"Kameron, these past few months, you haven't been the man I thought I knew," Michele started, "I wasn't feeling well, myself, and I didn't want to risk catching Covid."

"Oh... That's fair." Kameron stated with relief. "I'm sorry you weren't feeling well. But I'm even more sorry you didn't feel like you could share that with me." Kameron shook his head because it was becoming crystal clear that they were in a bad place.

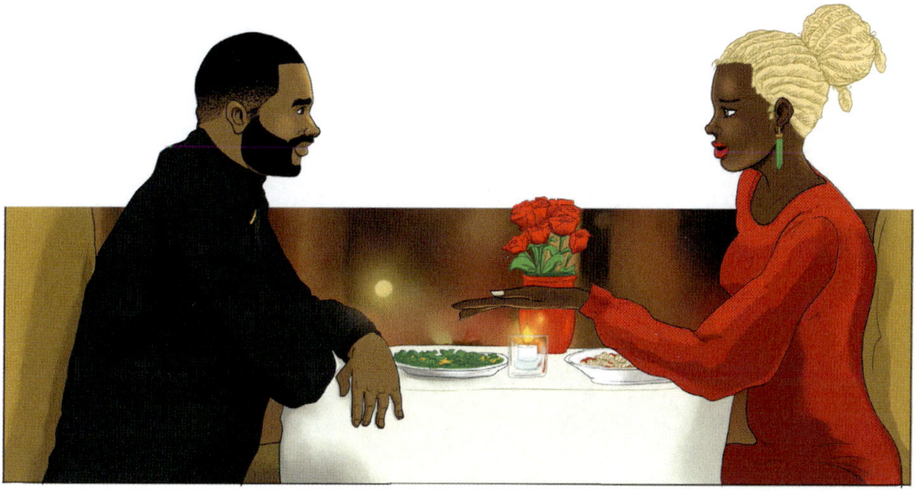

"Babe– Michele... I went with my Pops, Ven, and Van to the Rebalanced-Life Men's Health Center. While everyone else was doing their thing I decided to stop in to see the doctor, and–" Kameron's voice trailed off.

Michele's eyes widened. "Are you okay?"

"No. I think something's wrong," said Kameron, quietly, again regretting his choice of words at the table.

Michele felt hollow and shocked, still staring at him in concern.

"Wait, I mean... Something is wrong between us. This space we're in, right now." Kameron tried to clean up his previous choice of all-too-honest words.

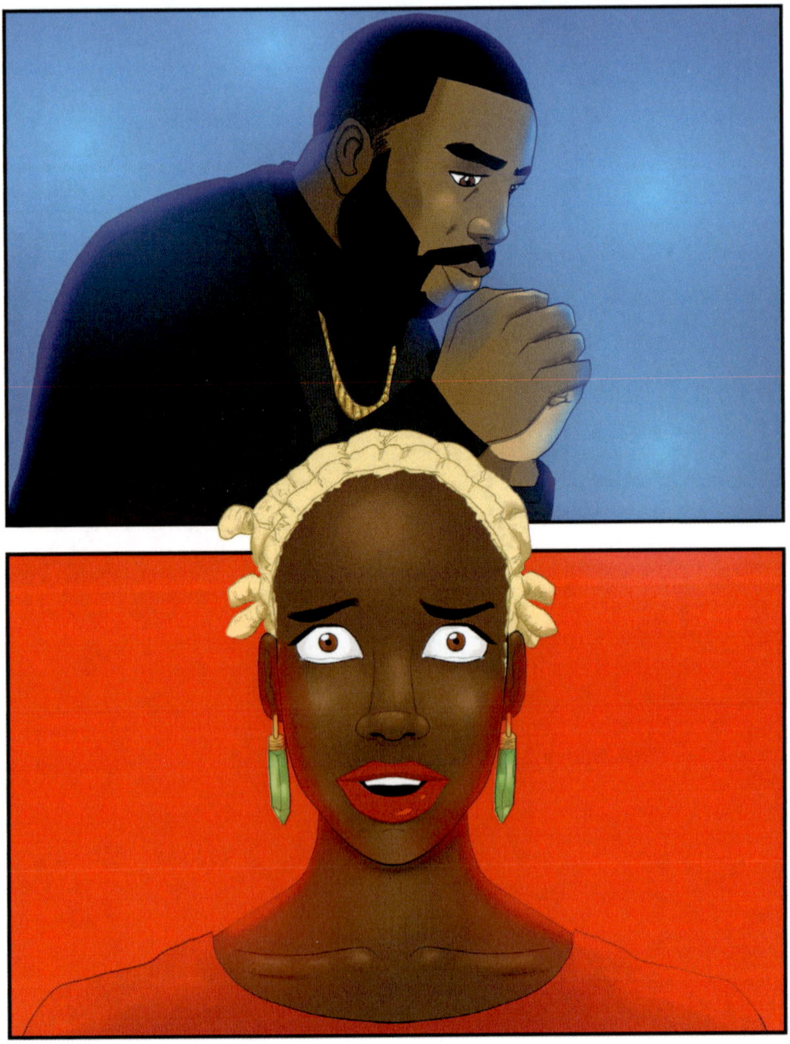

All of a sudden Michele came over and pulled Kameron in close. He embraced her and held on with his eyes closed as if eternity could fit within a minute. Her fragrance was sweet and alluring, and the touch of her body he had longed for felt like he was holding a brand-new version of her with a bonus any man would love. On the inside, he prayed he was the only man still loving it, for he was holding his greatest friend in life.

Michele fell apart in his arms, sobbing uncontrollably to his confusion.

Kameron did his best to be supportive as they sat back down, this time on the same side of the booth, as she continued to cry. He handed her a linen napkin from the table.

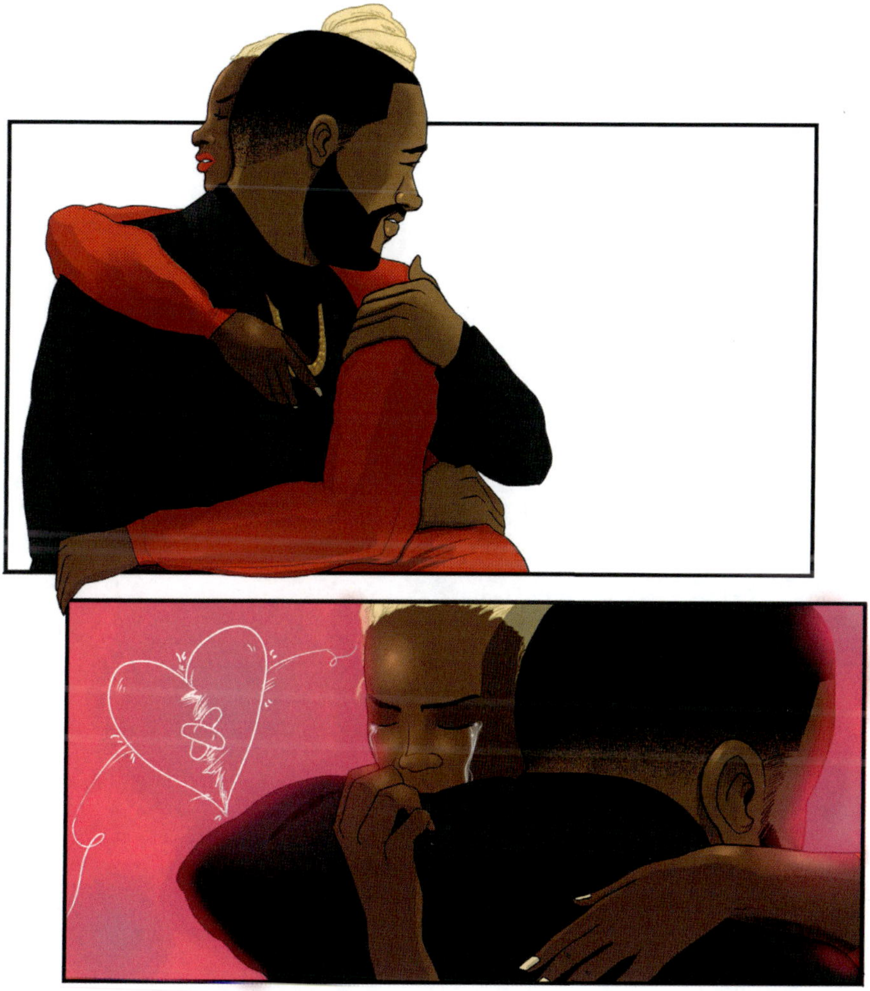

Finally, Michele regained her composure.

“I had all kinds of thoughts going through my head. I thought you moved on from us. You were so out of character and didn’t seem interested in me at all. I had to leave because I was so stressed and–”

Michele reached for Kameron’s hand and put it on her stomach.

“This was the main reason I didn’t come over when you were sick. I didn’t want to be pregnant with Covid,” Michele finally said the word out loud.

Kameron was overjoyed at the thought of finally being a dad. They had been trying to get pregnant for a year and a half. He remembered Pops’ wisdom about how a man can never truly be ready. He was excited, scared and overwhelmed all at the same time.

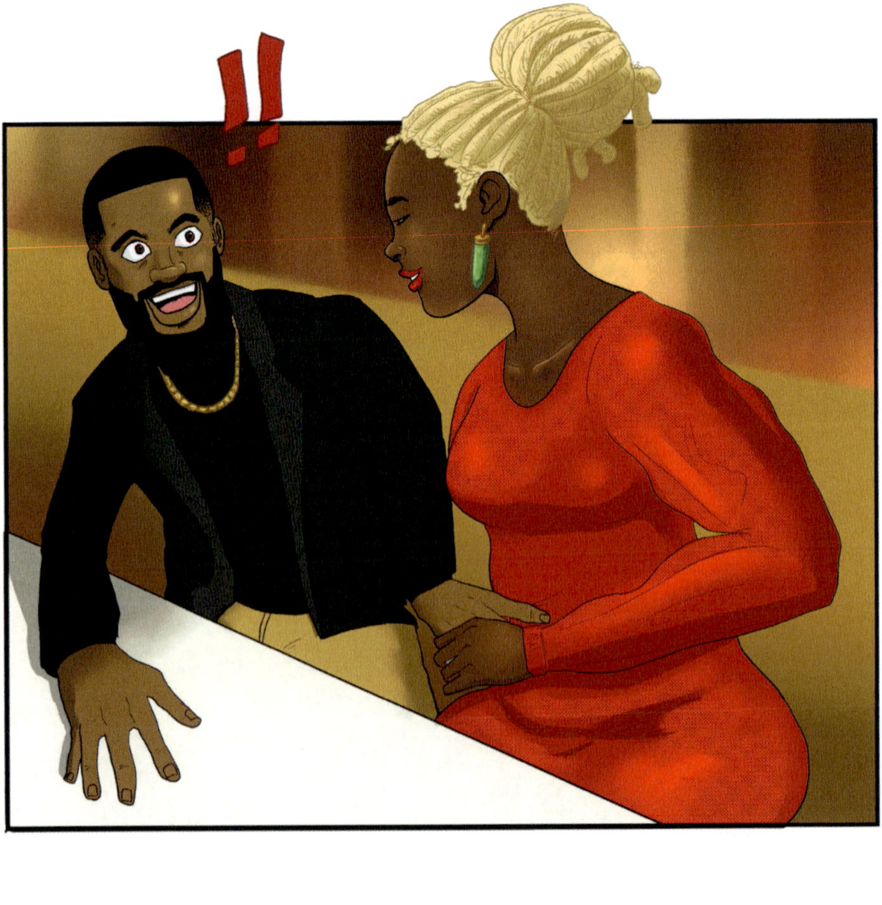

"Michele, I'm so happy. I want more than anything to celebrate this right now... but I originally asked you here to tell you that I took some tests while I was at the center. The doc asked me to come in so we can go over the results."

Kameron hated his luck at this moment. The absolute happiest time of his life and now he has these results looming over him. He saw the worry crease her brow. His hand on Michele's stomach in the booth became another full embrace of their bodies.

They sat in a mutually-understood pause of silence. To preserve the joy of the moment, they called for the check and did their best to not think about the visit to the doctor.

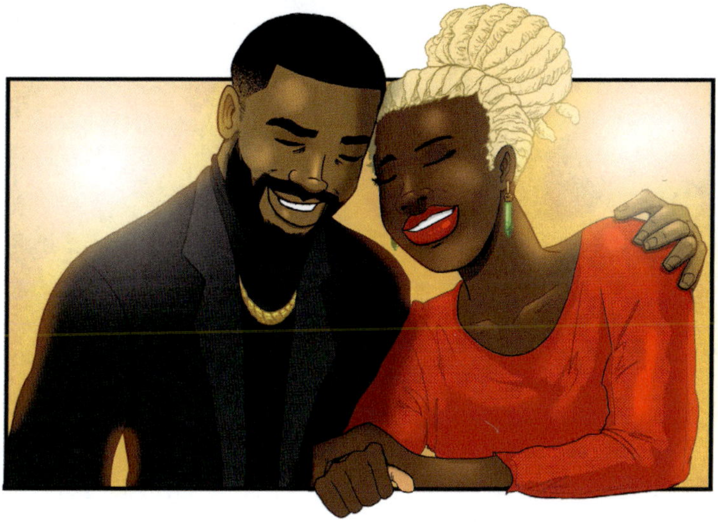

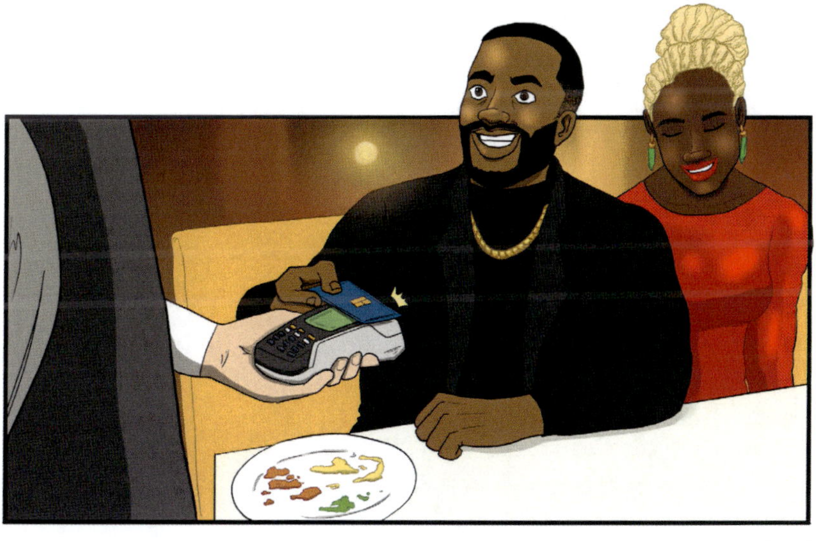

Lying in bed, holding one another past midnight at Kameron's place, they continued to focus on their growing family, ignoring the elephant in the room. King Kong was riding on its back in the corner like a Sleep Paralysis Demon, holding the test results.

Van and Ven popped up at the house the next morning. They were about to leave until they saw Michele's car in the driveway. Then it became a mission for intel. Kameron had been M.I.A. and they had to get the tea. They let themselves in his house and were shocked to see Kameron in the kitchen cooking breakfast and Michele sitting in the living room, kicked back with a three-month baby bump.

"Yo, what is this?" Van said with a smile from ear to ear.

"If I have to tell you then you have bigger problems than you realize," Michele said with a smile from ear to ear.

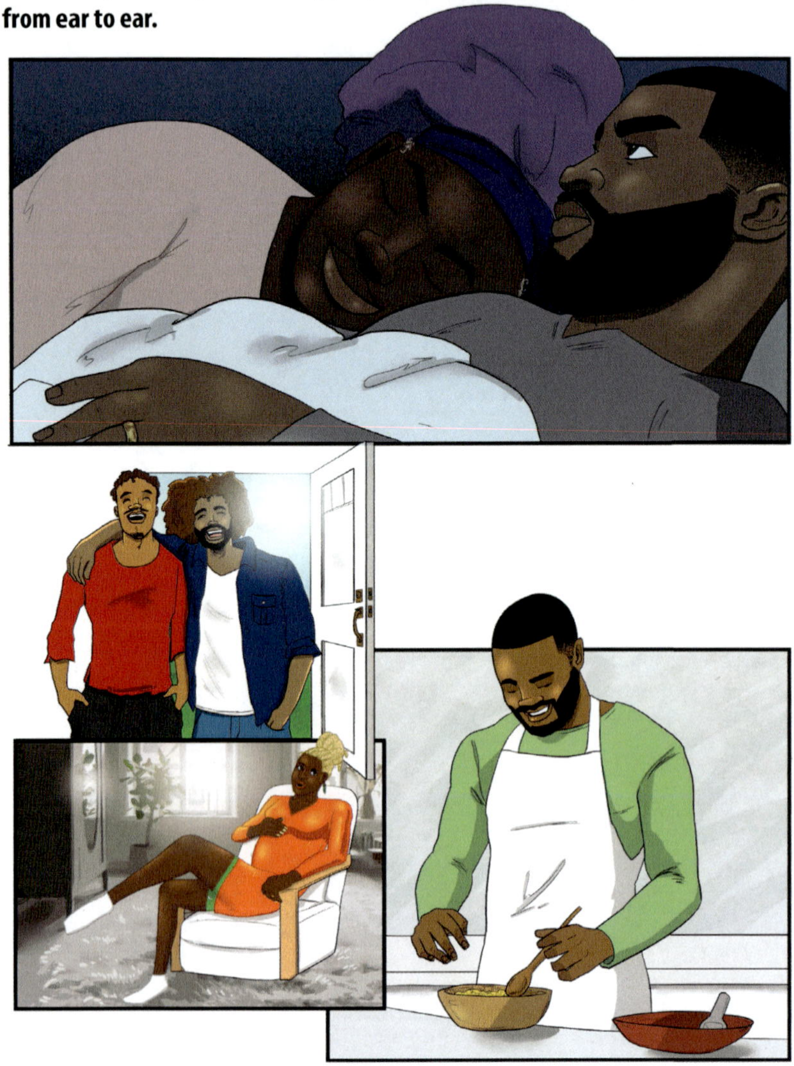

"Aaaahhhhwwww, snap!! Congratulations!" Ven said as he ran over to gently hug Michele.

They sat amongst each other in awe of the fact that their children would get to have the benefit of growing up together just like them. They talked about old times and how they would have to all get together to celebrate the next generation.

"But, Bro, what's really going on with you? I'm glad that you and Michele are vibing and for your, I mean our, newest family member-to-be but you have been acting hella weird lately," Van looked at Kameron with genuine concern in his gaze.

Ven was also looking intently at him. Kameron cleared his throat and Michele got off of the couch and put her hand on his shoulder to support him. Kameron slowly explained what he had been experiencing. He told Van and Ven that they had both been going through so much that he didn't want to burden them with what he was going through.

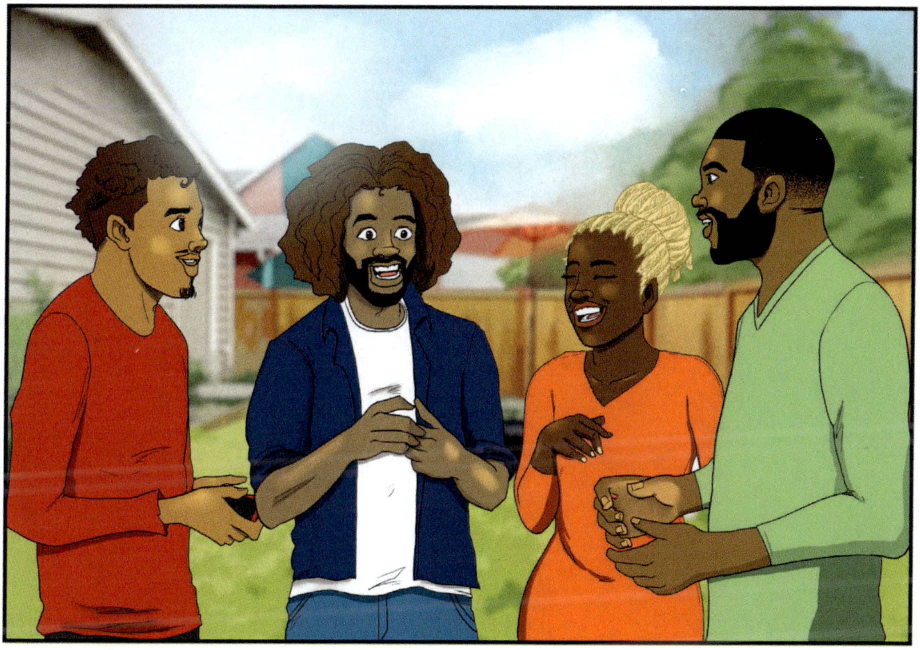

They all sat there at a loss for words. Michele kissed Kameron on the cheek and went upstairs to give them some time together. She knew that outside of herself and his own parents, there was no one she trusted more than Van and Ven to make sure Kameron had the love and support he needed. They were only cousins, but they were close like brothers from the same womb.

The three of them made plans to meet up at the Rebalanced Life Center to go to the doctor with Kameron. Michele offered to meet him after his appointment, but they convinced her that she should try not to get too stressed out and that they would call her immediately after.

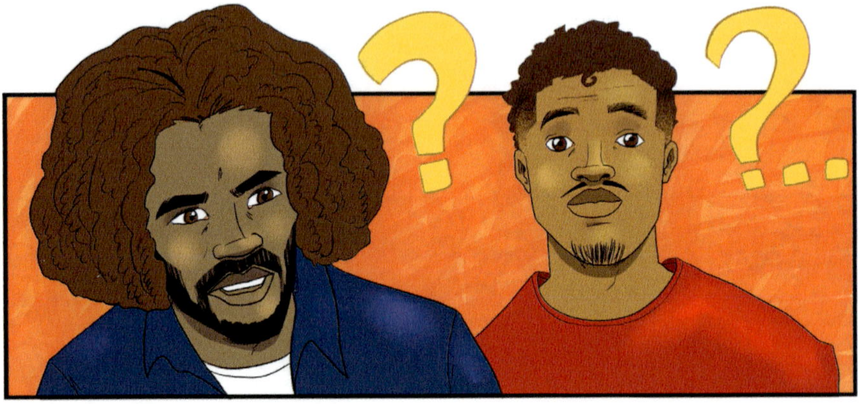

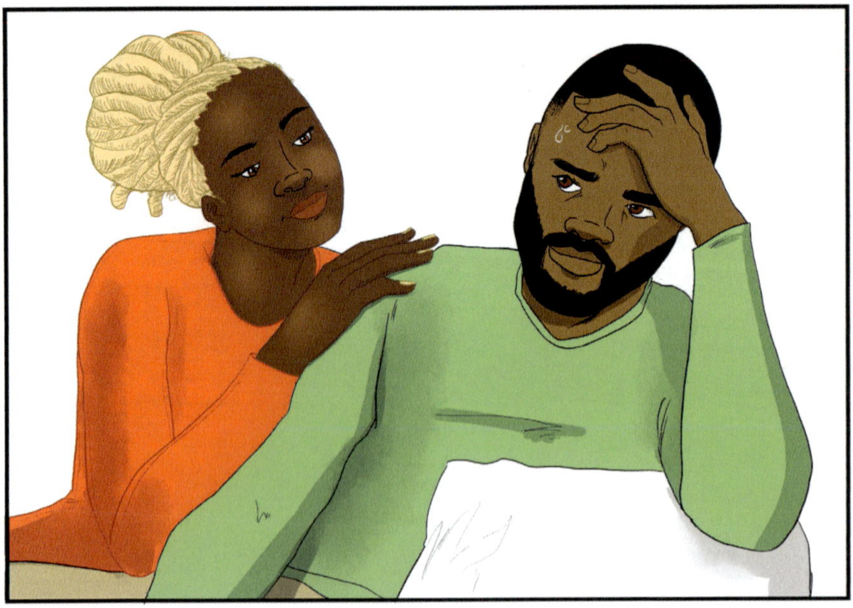

Once they arrived, Uncle Cooley was waiting for them. He popped Kameron in the back of the head.

"Boy, you're trying to have your mama kill both of us," He grabbed Kameron and hugged him tightly. They all went into the doctor's office with him when he was called.

"Well, Kameron, I first want to see how you are doing today and if it is okay to talk freely about your results?" The doctor asked him.

"Man, doc, these are my day ones. You can talk freely because they know where all the bodies are buried," Kameron said with humorous charm, trying his best to not let the intense worry creep into his voice.

"Kameron, some of the results are consistent with kidney disease. We need to run a few more tests to be 100% positive, but it is consistent with the test that we ran and your symptoms," The doctor's voice trailed off and he just scanned the room.

It was like the air was sucked out of the room for a full minute.

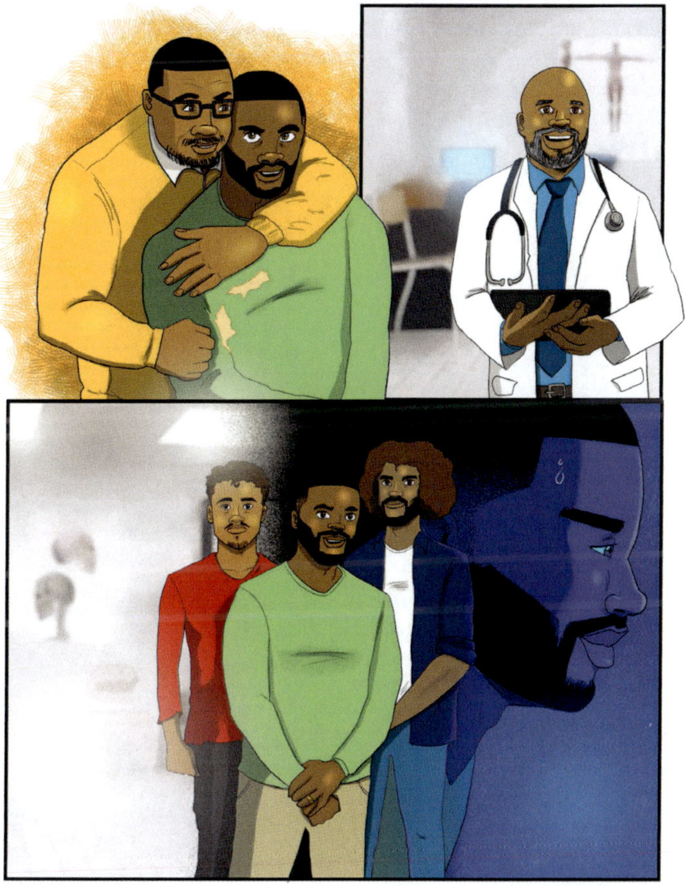

All of Kameron's guests stared in disbelief. The doctor restated his symptoms: nausea, vomiting, loss of appetite, fatigue, sleep problems, muscle cramps, swelling in his feet and ankles, decreased concentration and focus, and irritability. These were all signs of kidney disease.

"Doc, I need some time to process this and talk it over with my wife."
Breathless, Kameron had finally spoken. What was he going to tell Michele? What did all of this mean for his family-to-be? The doctor could tell he was spiraling again.

"Take your time, Kameron, but be sure not to take too long. There are still preventive measures we can take to avoid any further damage. Don't lose hope," he said with a hand to his shoulder.

Kameron hugged his people tightly and went home to share the diagnosis with Michele.

He felt horrible for putting all of this on her after everything they've struggled with, and now the pregnancy. He felt guilty and undeserving of love... and then she held him.

"Kam, look at me. We've gotten through everything else together...we'll make it through this, too." The embrace tightened and lasted a long while.

"Whether in sickness or in health, you will always have my love." Michelle kissed Kameron and his face lit up, remembering the day they promised that to each other at the altar.

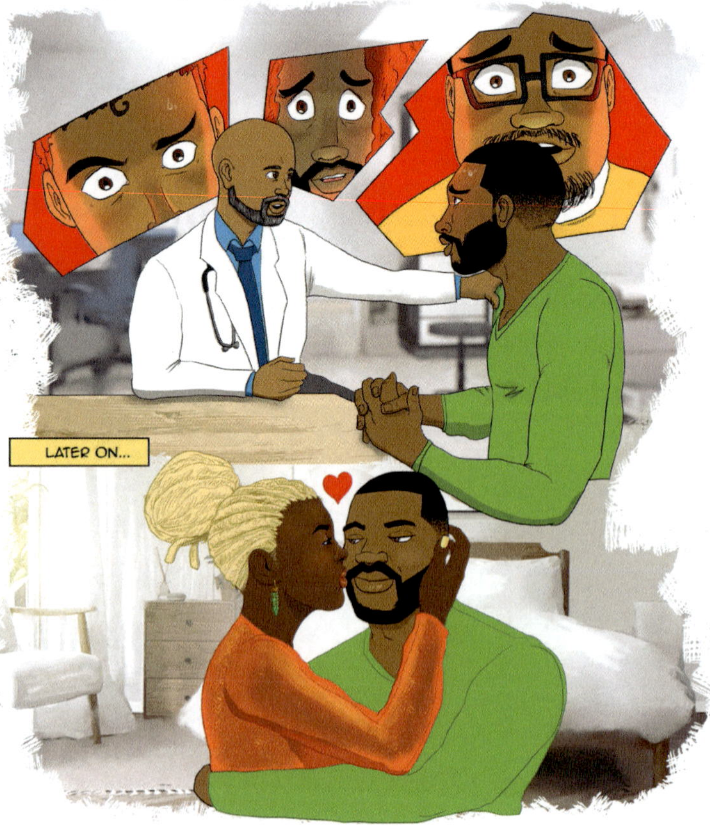

REFLECTION QUESTIONS

What were some of the symptoms of kidney disease Kameron experienced in the book?

Reflection Questions

What were some of the emotions Kameron experienced after he found out he had high kidney disease?

Reflection Questions

Can you relate to any of these emotions?

Reflection Questions

In the book, Kameron was nervous about his test results.
Have you ever experienced this?

Reflection Questions

Why do you think it's sometimes hard for men to prioritize their health?

What are ways to overcome this?

Reflection Questions

What was the role of Kameron's support system in helping him through this new experience?

Reflection Questions

Who is your support system?

Reflection Questions

When is the last time you had your kidneys checked?

Reflection Questions

When is your next doctor appointment?

Reflection Questions

What is one actionable step you can take this week to promote your personal health and wellbeing?

Made in the USA
Coppell, TX
21 June 2026

81339014R10026